YOGA FUN A-Z

Written by Joy Rush

Illustrated by Hannah Sprague

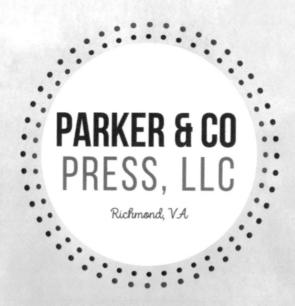

Published by Parker & Co., LLC
P.O. Box 50040
Richmond, VA 23250

ISBN: (paperback): 978-1-7363475-0-8
ISBN: (hardback): 978-1-7363475-1-5
ISBN: (ebook): 978-1-7363475-2-2

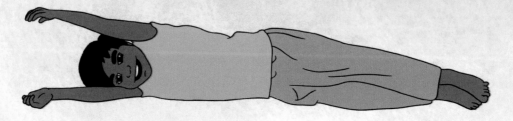

Dedication Page

TO MY SON,
Henry, thank you for being my number one fan in everything that I do.
Mommy loves you more than words can express.

TO MY GRANDMOTHER,
Evelyn, thank you for your encouragement and for showing me that life
is filled with unlimited opportunities to share my joy.

TO ALL MY LITTLE YOGIS AND YOGA FAMILIES,
Thank you for your continuous support. I have been inspired by so many
of you, and I hope you enjoy this work from my heart.

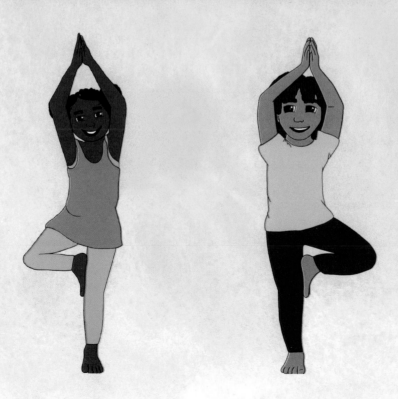

A FOR Alligator

Let's get started with a super fun pose! I lay flat on my belly with my head on my hands like an alligator hiding quietly - then "Chomp, Chomp, Chomp!" I open my arms and clap on each side. "WHAT FUN!"

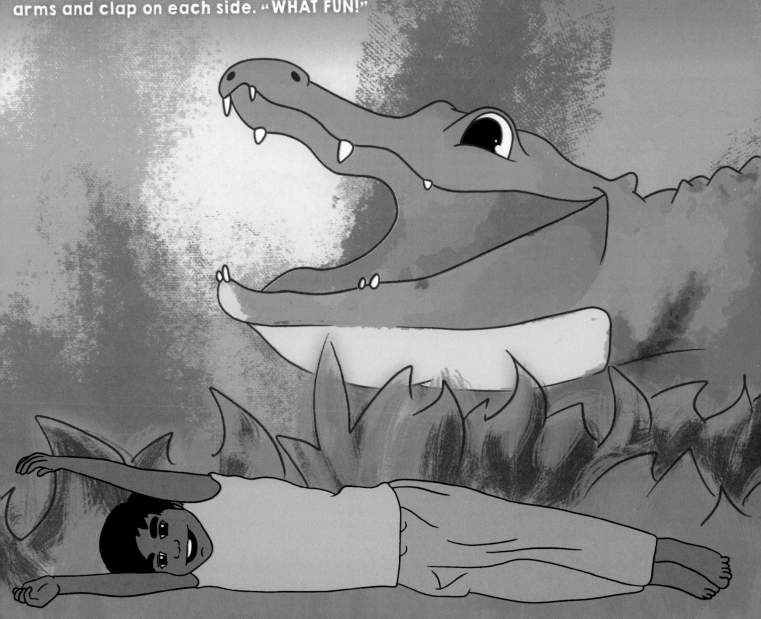

B FOR Balloon Breath

I sit on my bottom with both of my hands on my belly. I take a BIG breath in through my nose. I fill my belly just like air in a balloon and count 4, 3, 2, 1. "POP!" I blow out my air slowly imagining my balloon floating down to my hands "Whoooooo."

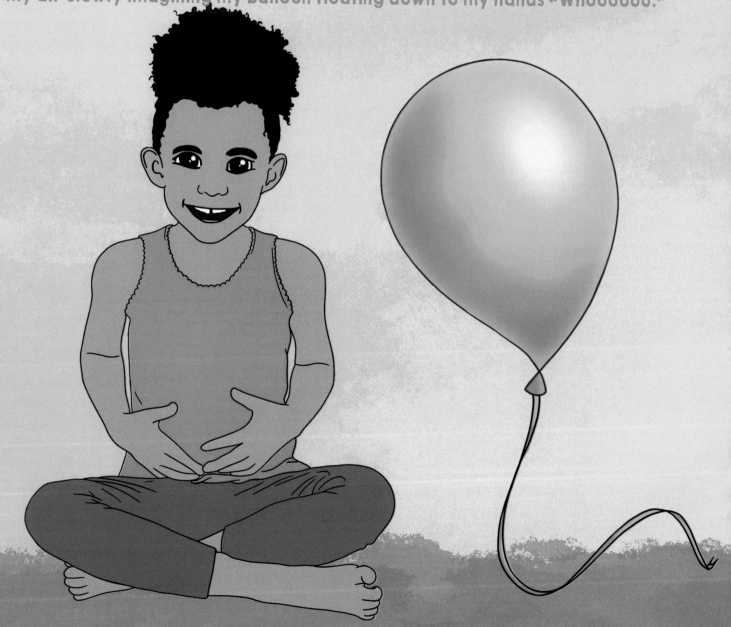

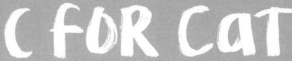

C FOR CAT

Just like a cat, I get on all fours. My knees are shoulder width apart and my hands are under my shoulders as I roll my back up towards the sky. I breathe in through my nose as I tuck my head towards my heart. As I breathe out, a soft "meow," I purr. I did Cat Pose!

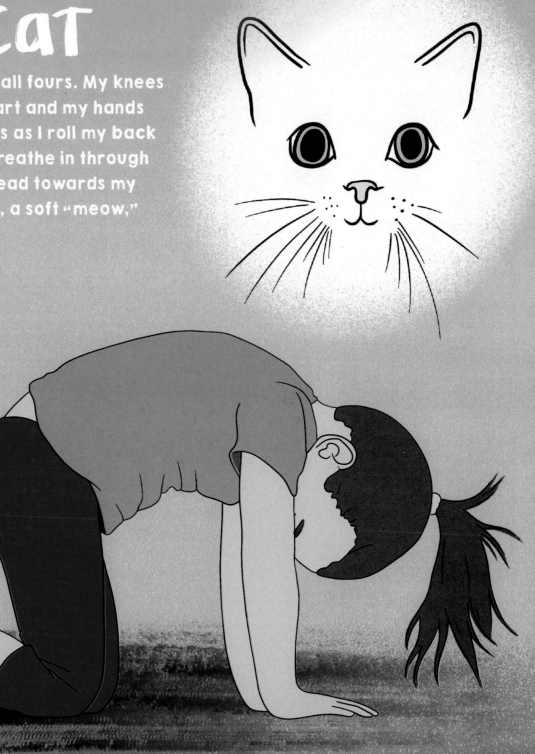

D FOR DOWNWARD DOG

I start on my hands and knees like Cat Pose with toes curled under. I straighten my legs and lift my hips up towards the sky. With my head relaxed between my arms, I can see the world from upside down! Oh, what YOGA FUN!

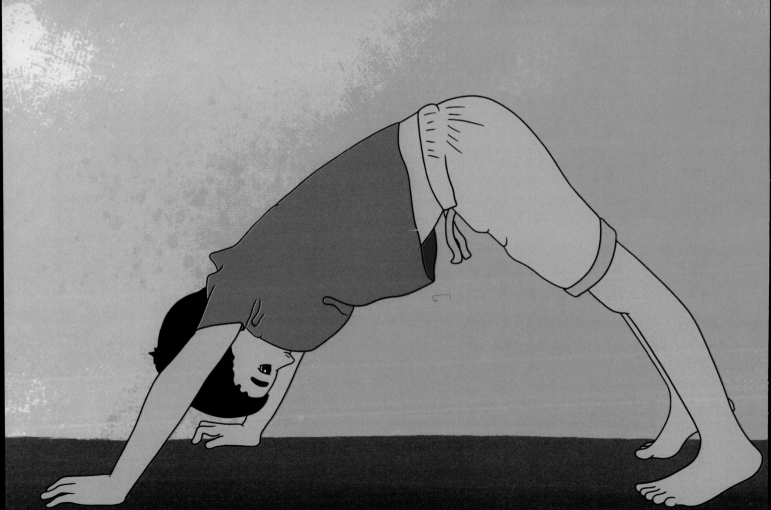

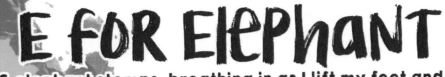

E FOR ELEPHANT

With BIG elephant stomps, breathing in as I lift my feet and out...STOMP, STOMP, STOMP, I stretch my arms above my head and make my trunk holding my hands together. Now, bending forward from my waist, I sway my trunk slowly from side to side - going UP and DOWN. Breathing big elephant breaths in through my nose and blowing out as I make my elephant trumpet sound.

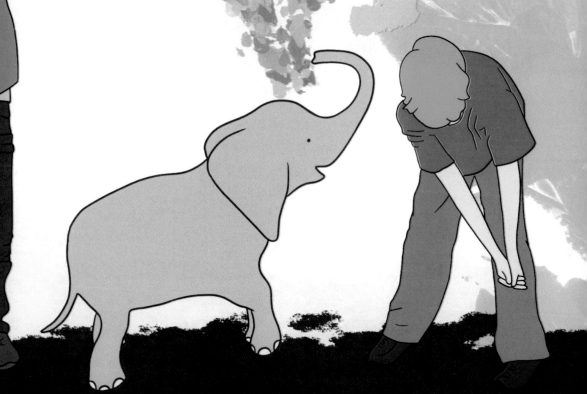

F FOR FLOWER

I love seeing flowers grow in spring; today a flower is what I will be. I sit down, bend my knees, put the bottoms of my feet together. I sit tall as I slide my hands under my ankles with my palms facing the sun. Now, I lift my legs and balance on my bottom. I wiggle my hands and feet, just like petals growing and flowing.

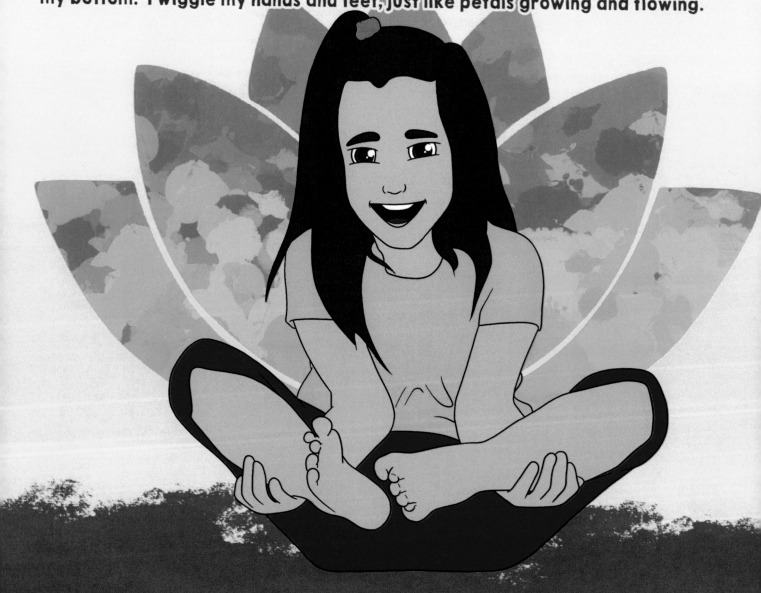

G FOR GIRAFFE

Giraffes are so cool and tall! With my legs shoulder-width apart, I stand tall, pushing one leg out like a lunge and the other slightly back. I stretch one hand above my head towards the sky imagining my long giraffe neck while the other hand drops behind my knee. I breathe in…and I breathe out. I am surrounded by beautiful safari trees.(Big yogis may know this pose as a reverse warrior.)

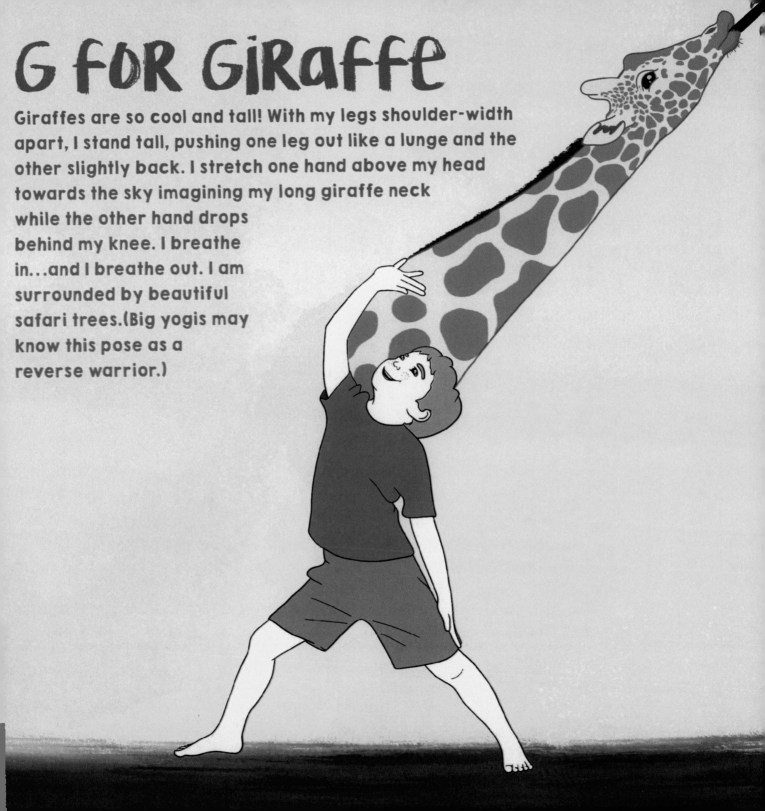

H FOR Happy Baby

Happy Baby Pose is so much FUN! I lie on my back and bring my knees toward my chest. I wiggle my feet a bit, point my toes towards the sun and grab the outside of my feet. I breathe in and out as I roll back and forth, "Happy Baby!"

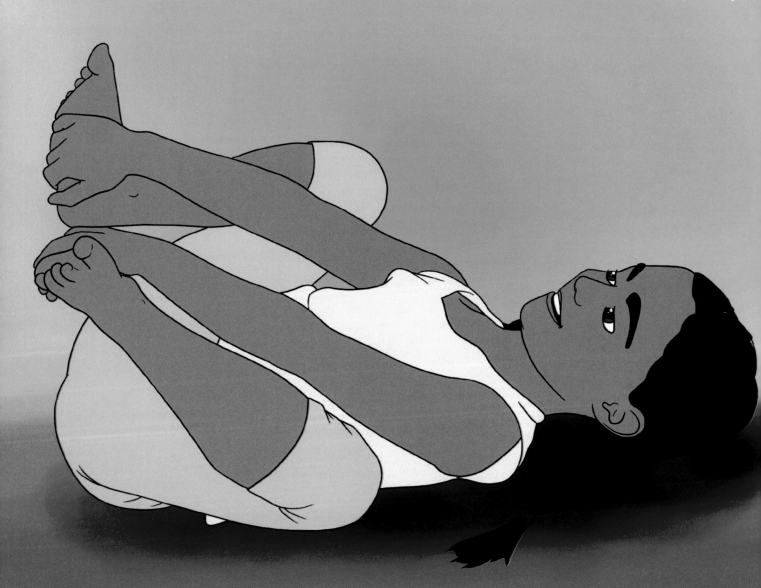

I FOR INHALE

Did you know there are different ways to inhale? You can breathe in through your nose or your mouth, slow or quick, short or long. Let's try a few. I take a quick breath in through my nose…and release. Now, try a long deep breath. I breathe in through my nose, count to 4 and blow it out slowly through my mouth….
"Wheeew!" Making a sound like the wind! There is bunny breath too and so much more! Let's try one more, take three quick bunny breaths in and three quick breaths out. Can you wiggle your nose like a bunny? That's funny.

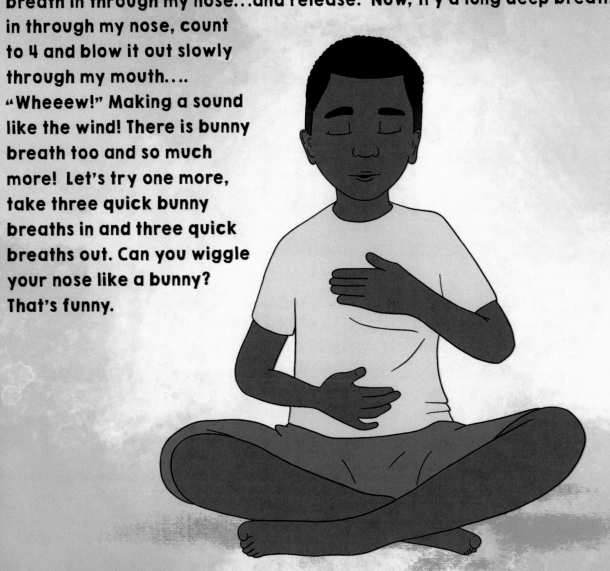

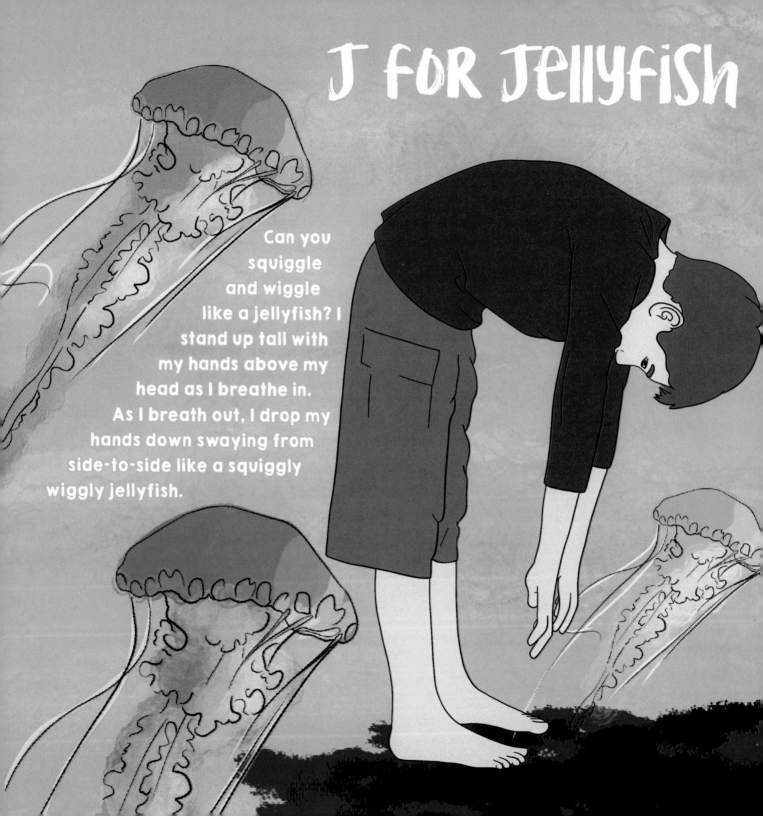

J FOR JellyfiSh

Can you squiggle and wiggle like a jellyfish? I stand up tall with my hands above my head as I breathe in. As I breath out, I drop my hands down swaying from side-to-side like a squiggly wiggly jellyfish.

K FOR KITE

Let's be a kite, flying in the wind! I balance on one foot like the kite string. I put my hands above my head as I breathe in swaying to the left and breathe out swaying to the right.

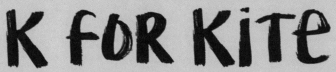

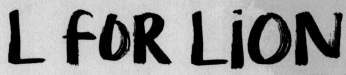

L FOR LiON

Lion is the king of the jungle.
I get on my knees, open my
mouth wide, stick out my
tongue and
"Rrrrrrrrrrrrr!" That
was FUN! How loud
was your roar?

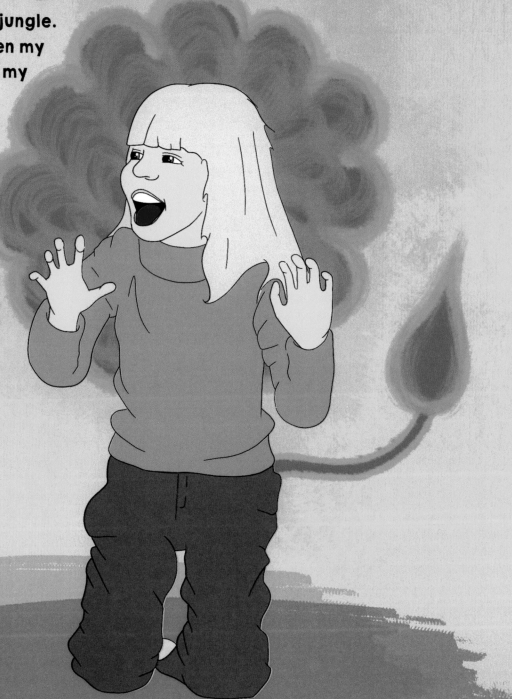

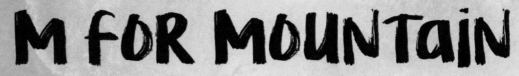

M FOR MOUNTAIN

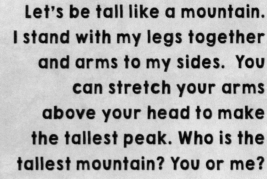

Let's be tall like a mountain. I stand with my legs together and arms to my sides. You can stretch your arms above your head to make the tallest peak. Who is the tallest mountain? You or me?

N FOR NAMASTE

Namaste is my favorite greeting of all. Whether we sit or stand, I place my hands together before we part ways. What does it mean to me, you ask? The peace in me sees the peace and kindness in you too!

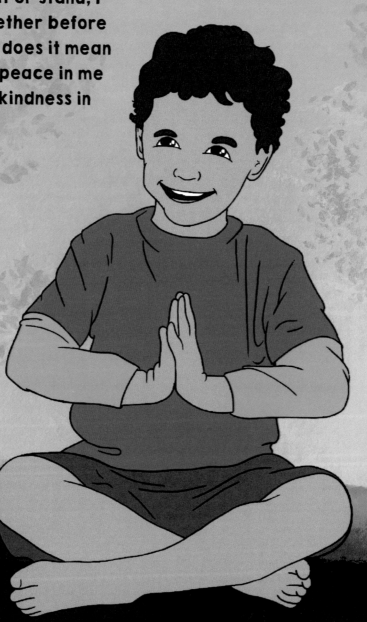

O FOR OCTOPUS

Let's use our imagination as we dive deep into the ocean blue. I lay gently on my back, float my arms and legs all the way up. As I float about, I sway my arms and legs from side-to-side, a little wiggly just like a squiggly swimming octopus.

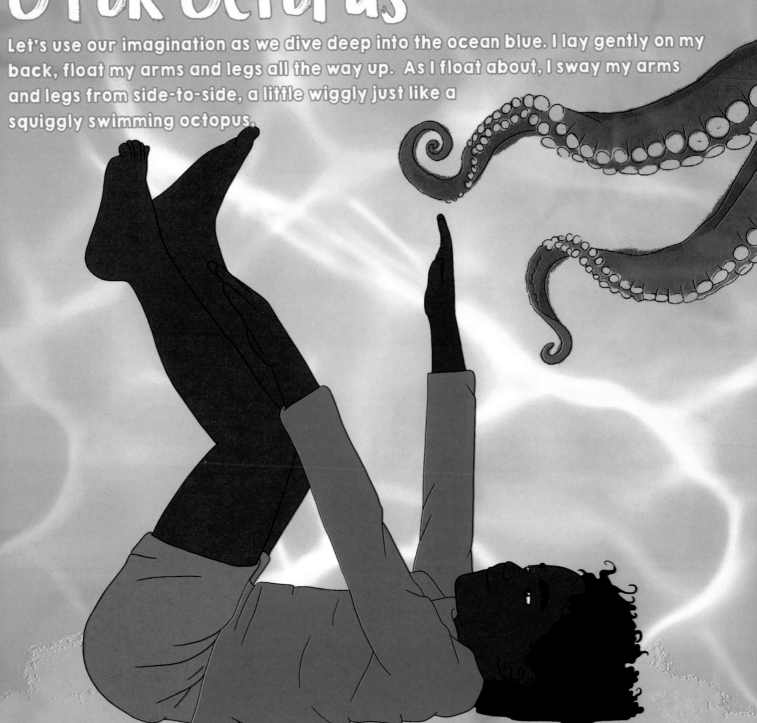

P FOR PLANE

I stand tall with my head held high, then stretch my arms out on each side. As I get ready for take-off, I lift one leg up and lean forward...Up, Up and away we go! Flying high in the sky, swaying from left to right.

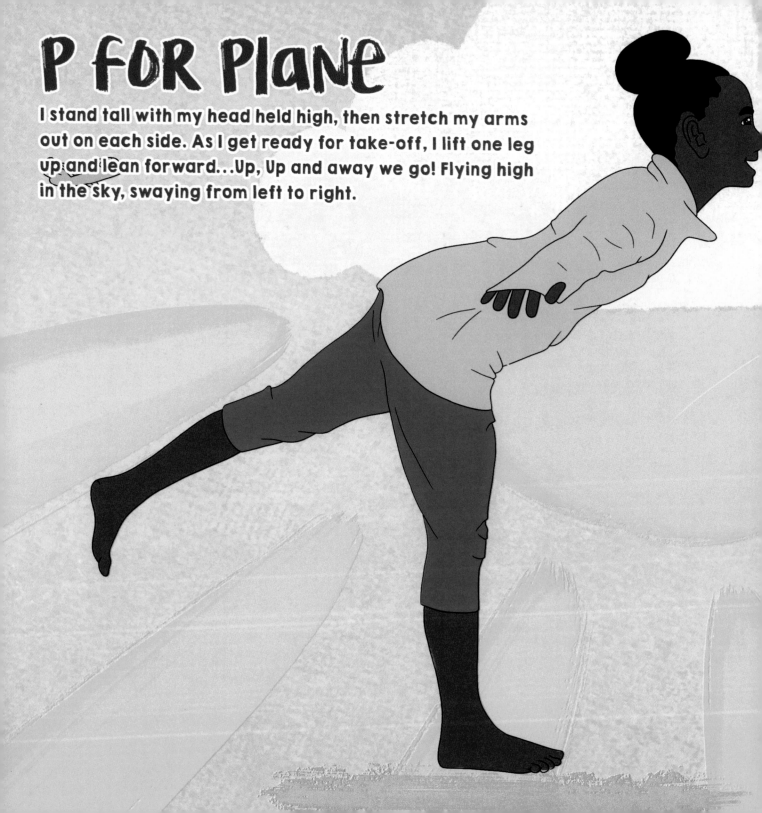

Q FOR QUIET TIME

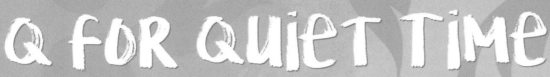

Quiet time is a super special time of day. It's time to relax from my head to my feet. I sit on my yoga mat or even my bed, to find my calm. I breathe in through my nose and count...I, 2,3,4, then breathe out slowly like the wind...I, 2, 3, 4. On days when I have butterflies in my tummy or feel silly in my brain, quiet time helps me feel calm and happy.

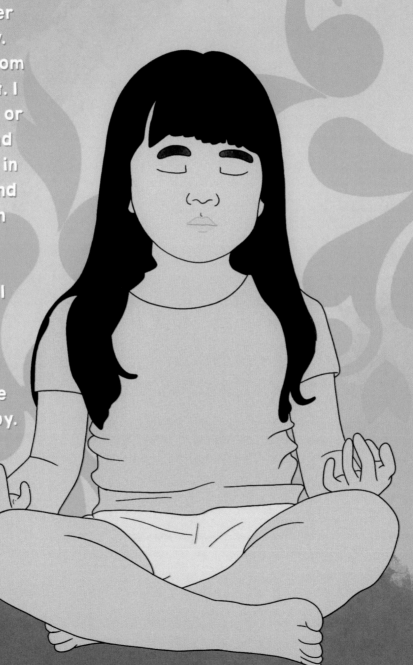

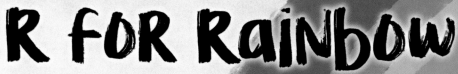

R FOR Rainbow

I raise my hands above my head and press my hands together. Slowly bending to one side of my rainbow and then the other. Rainbows are filled with magic and you are too!

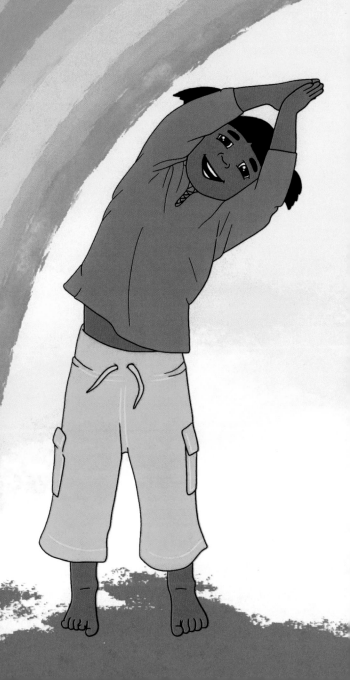

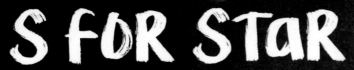

S FOR STAR

Stars twinkle high in the night's sky.
I'm going to be a star tonight. I
stretch my arms and legs out wide.
I sparkle even brighter by wiggling

my fingers and even my
toes, as I breathe in and
breathe out. Have you ever
seen a star so bright?

T FOR Table

It's picnic time and I'll be table! I sit with my legs stretched out, then bend my knees and put my feet flat on the floor. My hands are on the floor too, right behind me. I push my belly up and flat as a table top. I am strong! Can you balance an apple on your belly?

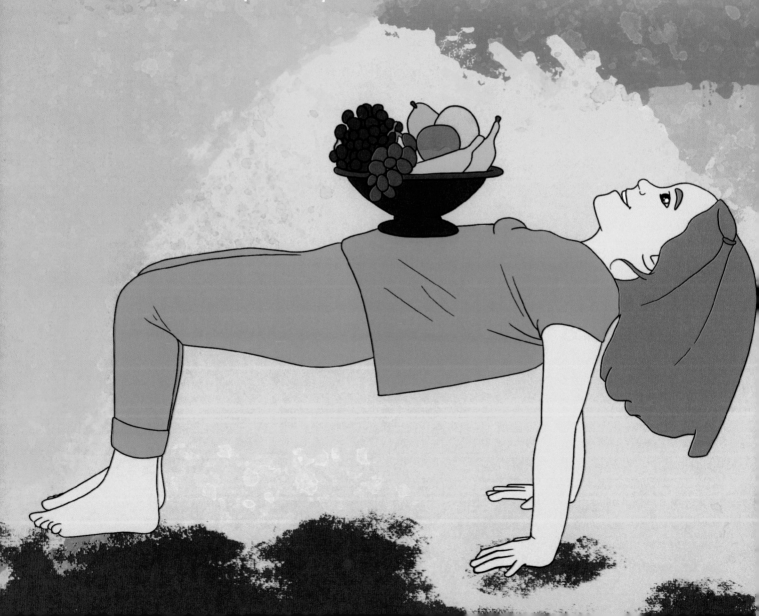

U FOR UNICORN

Standing with my feet together, sliding one leg over the other.
I cross my arms to make my unicorn horn…and "Neighhh!"
I dash off leaving trails of magic behind me.

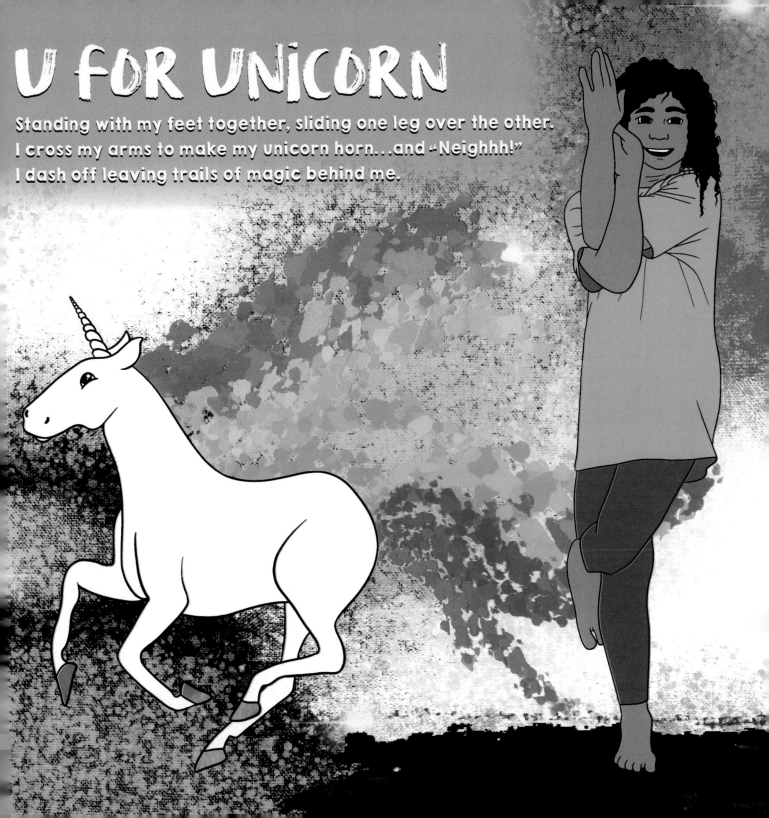

V FOR VOLCANO

Standing tall like the tallest volcano with my feet together and my hands at my side, I stand still quietly breathing in through my nose and slowly out. I listen for a rumble of the lava below....then all of a sudden, ERUPT! I jump my legs out on each side with hands above my head. I am a VOLCANO!

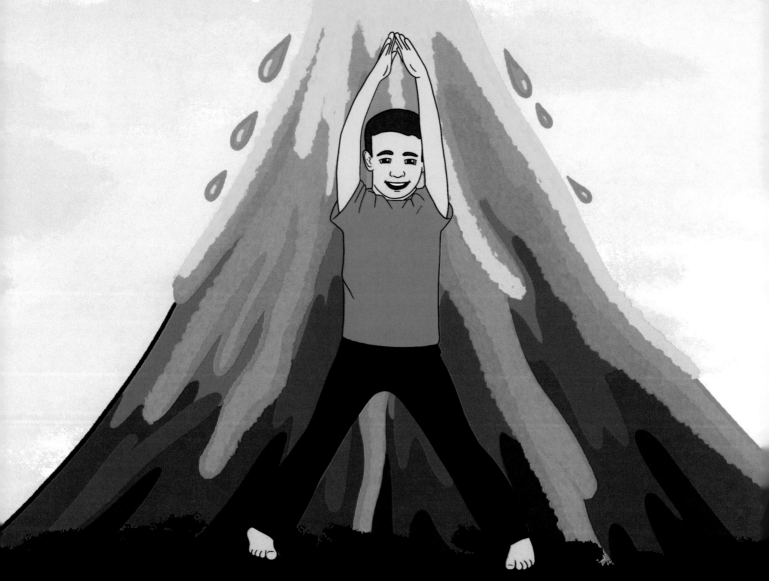

W FOR WARRIOR

As a warrior, I am strong! I stand with my feet apart and my arms stretched out wide. My hands are faced down towards the earth. I point one foot to the side with a bent knee and I breathe in 1, 2, 3, 4 and out 1, 2, 3, 4. I am the greatest warrior because I am me!

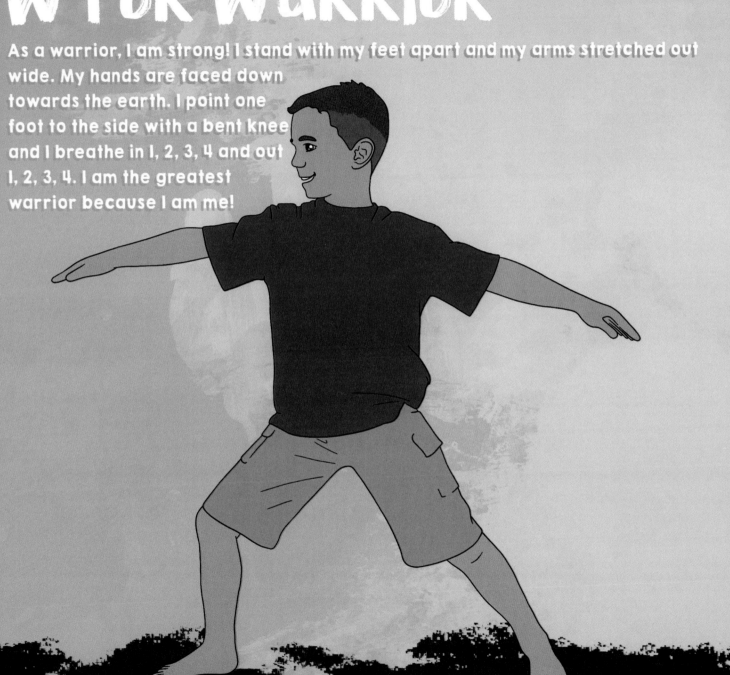

X FOR LETTER X

Let's have some fun with the alphabet. I stand with my feet together and my hands by my sides. Now here comes the big surprise... let's jump out with our hands in the air and our feet apart. Can you see what I am? I'm the Letter X!

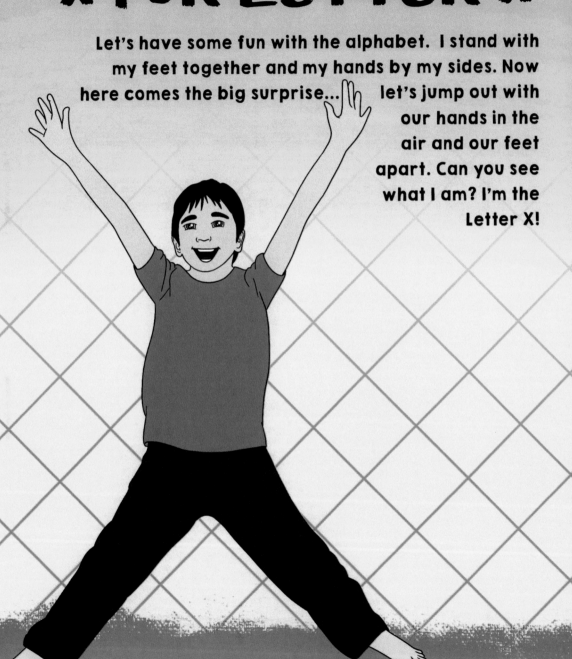

Y FOR YOU

Now it's your turn to pick a pose! Whether it's a mountain, a rainbow or even a star...it's yours to choose! Remember everything you do on one side, be sure to do on the other! Don't forget to breathe.

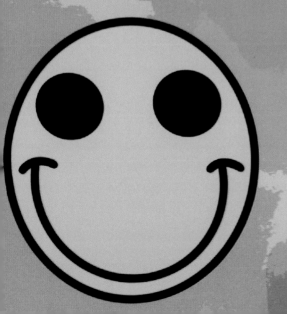
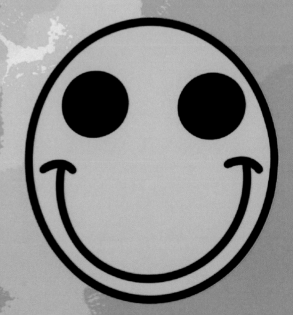

Z FOR ZERO

So much yoga fun, from A to Z. Now, we're at the end, there's zero to go...so zero is what I will be. I sit down with my legs crossed, stretch my hands all the way up and round to make a great big zero!

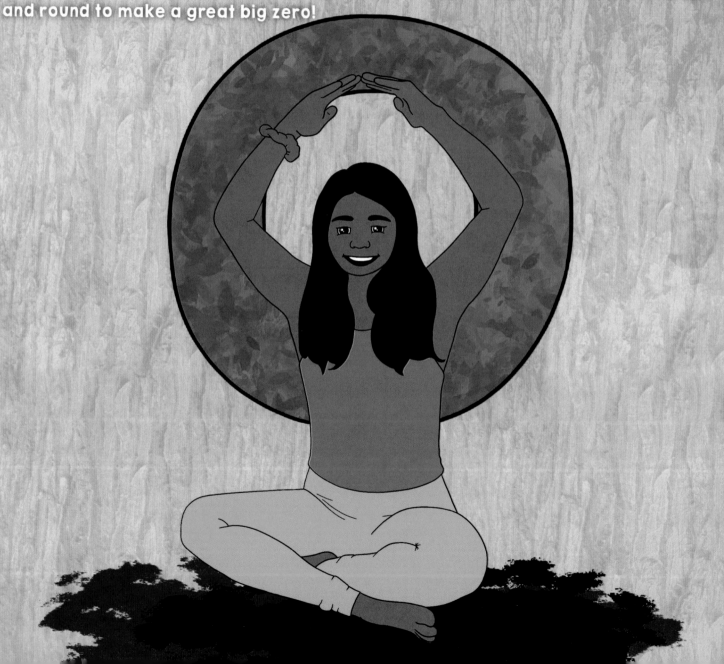

PARTNER POSES

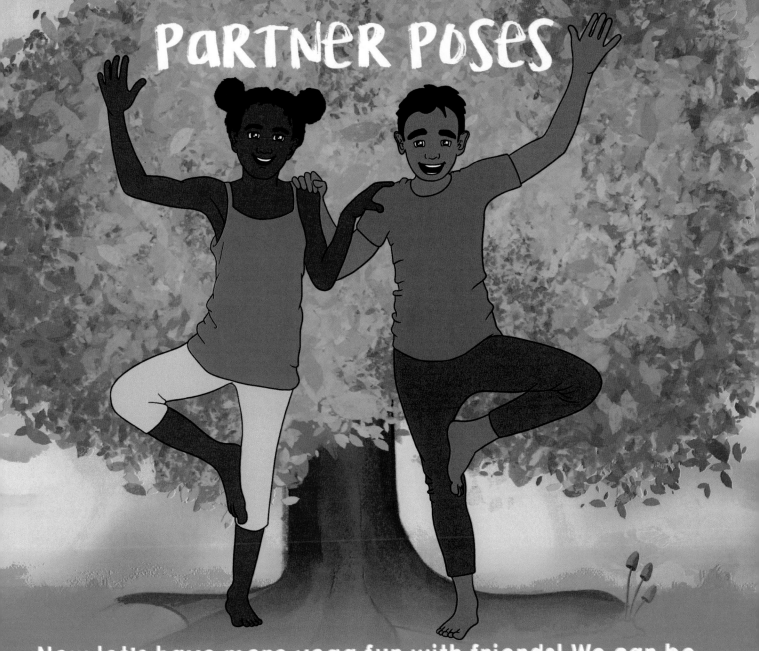

Now let's have more yoga fun with friends! We can be tall as a TREE. With my foot flat along my leg above or below my knee, I put one hand high like branches and the other shoulder-to-shoulder, you see. It's Tree Pose with you and me!

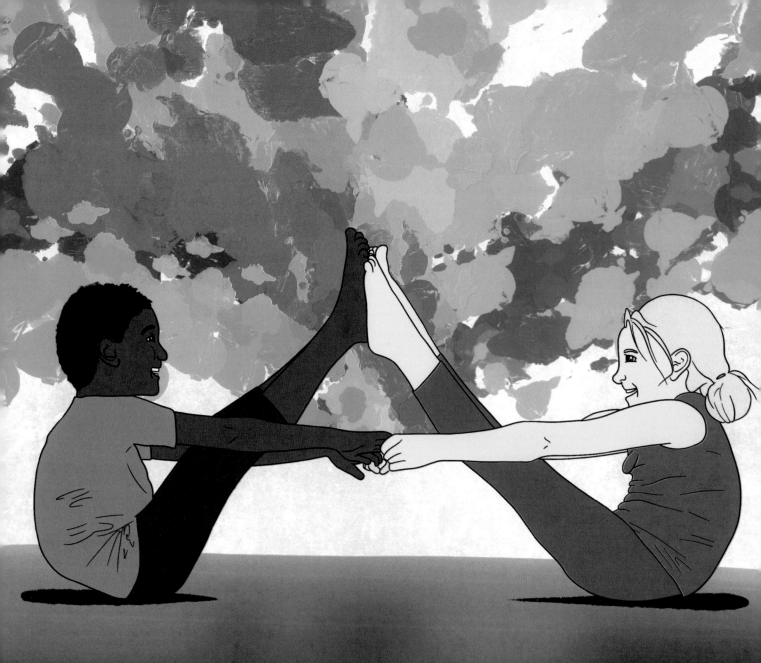

We can be a BOAT floating along in the river. Facing each other, hands-to-hands and feet-to-feet, we slowly raise our legs balancing with each other. We are a boat, you

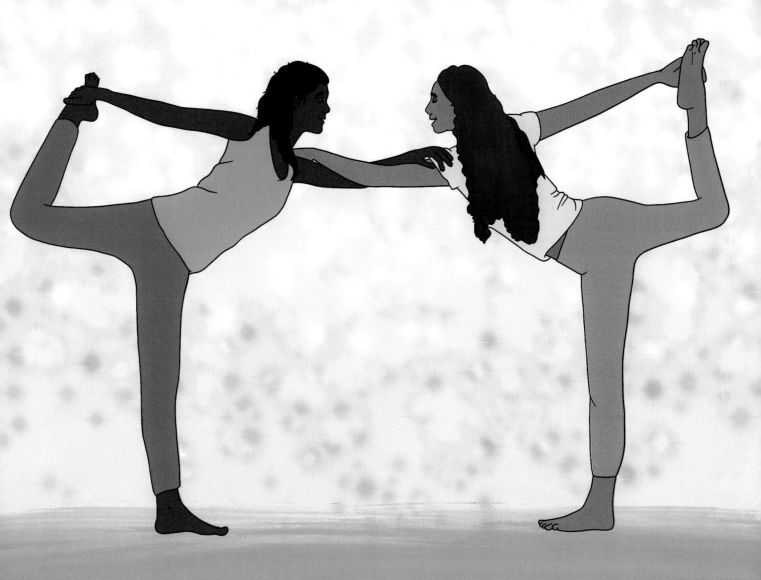

Let's dance together! Dancer Pose is fun with a
friend and easier too! Facing each other with hands
on each other's shoulder, we gently lift our legs by
holding the inside of our feet. Lift, lift and slowly
bend towards each other for a nice long stretch.
Yayyy, it's a dancer's duo with you and me! Now we
slowly place our legs back down. Let's do it again!

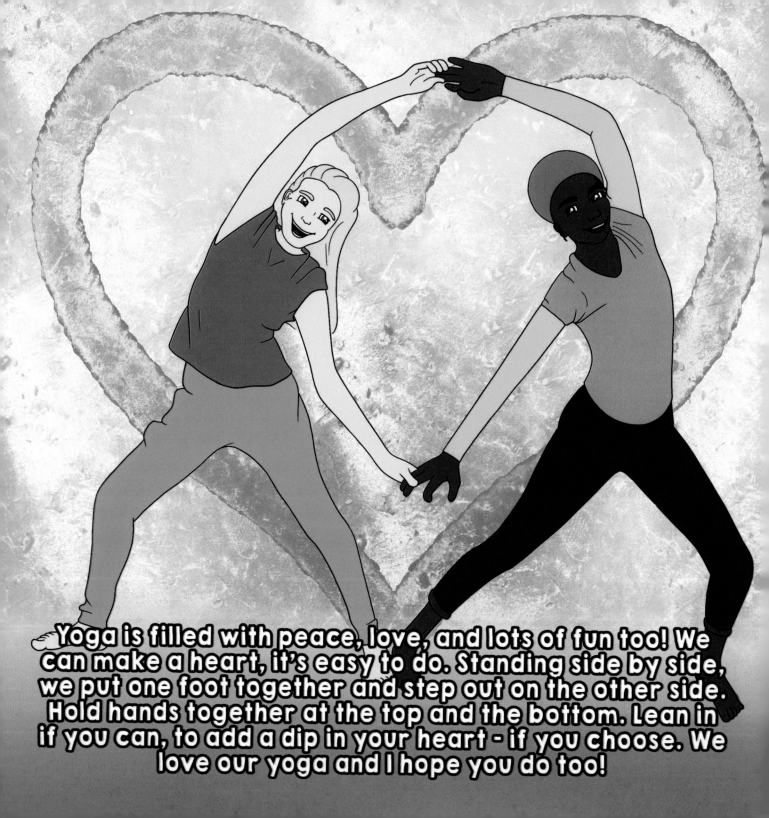

Yoga is filled with peace, love, and lots of fun too! We can make a heart, it's easy to do. Standing side by side, we put one foot together and step out on the other side. Hold hands together at the top and the bottom. Lean in if you can, to add a dip in your heart - if you choose. We love our yoga and I hope you do too!

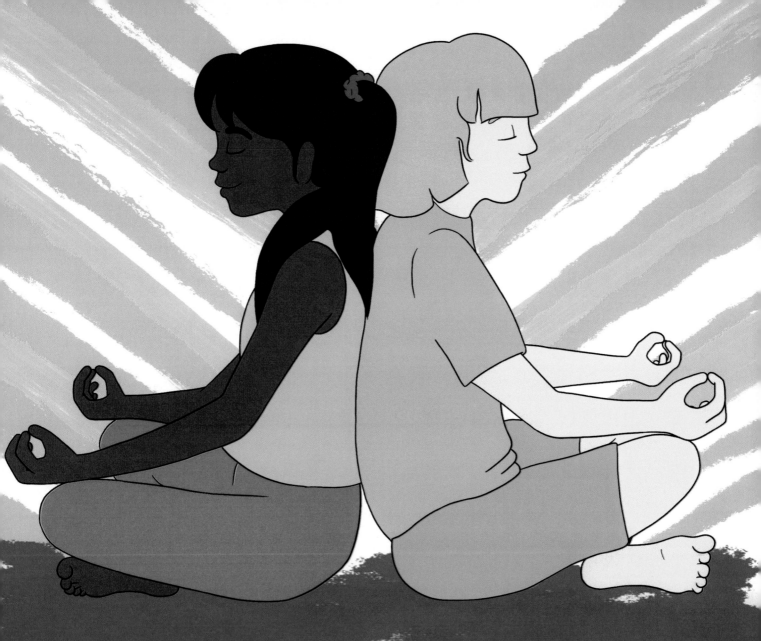

We can meditate together, did you know? Back to back as we breathe in...1, 2, 3, 4 and breathe out...1, 2, 3, 4. I place my hands on my knees and we can even say together "Peace begins with me."

Author's Bio:

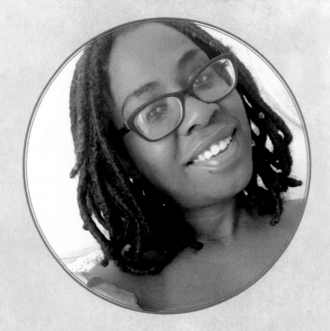

A native of Richmond, Virginia, Joy Rush is the owner of YOGA JOY Kids Studio, now an online kids yoga platform for children and families. A certified kids yoga instructor, Joy aims to introduce yoga, meditation, and mindfulness to children of all ages. With a goal to fill the diversity gap, Joy features children from all different ethnicities and backgrounds in her work. Joy has quickly become a leader in her field with sponsored YOGA JOY online programs all over the country. As the mother of one son, Henry, Joy enjoys spending quality time with her family, mentoring, and traveling the world.

www.yogajoyrva.com

BReathe in
as my hands go up!
BReath out as my hands
go down. I can be a
mountain. I can be a
staR. I can be Rainbow
high in the sky. Yoga
FUN FOR EVERYONE!

Made in the USA
Middletown, DE
10 May 2021